CHLORELLA:

The Ultimate Green Food

Nature's Richest Source of
Chlorophyll, DNA & RNA

A Health Learning Handbook

Beth M. Ley, Ph.D.

BL Publications
Detroit Lakes, MN

BL Publications, Detroit Lakes, MN
1-877-BOOKS11/www.blpublications.com
email: blpub@tekstar.com

Library of Congress Cataloging-in-Publication Data

Ley, Beth M., 1964-
  The ultimate green food : nature's richest source of chloro-phyll, DNA & RNA : a health learning handbook / Beth M. Ley.
      p. cm.
  ISBN 1-890766-28-3
  1. Chlorella as food. 2. Chlorella. 3. Chlorella--Therapeutic use.
I. Title.

  TX402.L493 2003
  641.3--dc22

                                    2003015456

Printed in the United States of America

This book is not intended as medical advice. Its purpose is solely educational. Please consult your healthcare professional for all health problems.

YOU NEED TO KNOW...
THE   HEALTH   MESSAGE

Do you not know that you are God's temple and that God's Spirit dwells in you? If anyone destroys God's temple, God will destroy him, For God's temple is holy and that temple you are. *1 Cor. 3:16-17*

So, whether you eat or drink, or whatever you do, do all to the glory of God. *1 Cor. 10:31*

Table of Contents

Introduction

Chlorella is a single-celled fresh-water, microscopic green algae, which provides a very well-balanced package of essential nutrients. Along with its rich stores of complete protein, Chlorella also provides essential fatty acids, carbohydrates, minerals, vitamins, enzymes, chlorophyll, RNA/DNA, antioxidants, special fiber and its own unique Chlorella Growth Factor (CGF). Working to maintain bodily health, prevent disease, and enhance recuperation, Chlorella can be thought of as a complete health supplement. It is truly the ultimate green food. Chlorella is so complete that we could survive on it alone for an extended period of time and in fact, NASA researchers have investigated this very possibility for astronauts in space travel.

Chlorella benefits us in four main ways:

1. **Provides complete nutrition to normalize body function**

2. **Supports and strengthens the immune system**

3. **Detoxifies and purifies the body**

4. **Promotes healthy cellular growth and repair to slow down aging**

A Brief History

Chlorella is one of the oldest forms of plant life on earth. It has the highest chlorophyll content of any known plant and this gives Chlorella its characteristic deep green color. The name Chlorella is derived from the Latin "chlor" for green and "ella" for small.

Even though Chlorella has existed on earth since its beginning, and was discovered in 1890 by a Dutch microbiologist named M. W. Beijerinck, Chlorella was not studied closely until the 1940s. Professor Beijerinck was the first to culture Chlorella in his laboratory.

Japan became the first world pioneer in developing the technology to commercially produce Chlorella. Chlorella has a tough outer cell wall making the nutrients inside the cell virtually inaccessible. This problem was overcome by a Japanese company who developed a unique process to break down the cell wall, while preserving the nutritional value contained within.

Today, Chlorella is cultivated in filtered fresh water ponds. With the favorable conditions of strong sunlight, pure water and clean air, the remarkable algae multiplies at an incredible rate, reproducing four times about every 20-24 hours.

Chlorella has many clinically-proven health benefits. Long acclaimed for its health promoting properties, Chlorella is highly regarded and well known throughout Japan. It is believed to be their #1 health food supplement with over 10 million people in Japan taking it regularly. In fact, more people in Japan take Chlorella than North Americans take Vitamin C - our most popular vitamin. Chlorella, dubbed the "Green Gem of the Orient," is deserving of its reputation as the ultimate green food.

In Japan, Chlorella is actually regarded as a functional whole food, rather than a dietary supplement. Functional foods are used mainly to nourish the human body after physical exertion, as a preventive measure against ailments and to promote longevity and vitality.

The popularity of Chlorella is quickly increasing in the United States. People are discovering that living in a world bombarded by chemicals and pollutants is disrupting the balance in our bodies, compromising our immune systems, decreasing our energy levels, clogging our organs, creating stress from head to toe, and increasing our risk of every kind of disease. As a true whole superfood, Chlorella has the tremendous ability to detoxify, energize, nourish and ultimately balance all of the body's systems for optimal function.

Chlorella: The Basics

Chlorella is a single-celled fresh-water, microscopic algae, measuring between 2 and 8 microns in diameter (1 micron is 1,000th of 1 millimeter). Chlorella cells are round in shape and almost the same size as human red blood corpuscles.

Scientifically, Chlorella belongs to green micro algae. The two most common strains are Chlorella pyrenoidosa and Chlorella vulgaris. They are very similar and for the purposes of this book, can be considered the same. Other relatives of the Chlorella family are ao-nori and kelp-like Wakame and Kombu which are also popular as food products.

The "green algae" is the most diverse group of algae, with more than 7,000 species growing in a variety of habitats. Like plants, green algae contain two forms of chlorophyll, which they use to capture light energy to fuel the manufacture of sugars, but unlike plants they are primarily aquatic. Because they are aquatic and manufacture their own food, these organisms are called "algae."

Chlorella is Single-celled Micro Algae

Unlike most plants of multi-cells, Chlorella is unicellular, which means each cell is a self-sufficient organism. Though we cannot tell by the naked eye, each Chlorella cell has its own organs and functions to live alone.

Chlorella is Very Productive

There are two types of reproduction for plants and animals; Asexual and unisexual. Chlorella is asexual. A 3 micron size Chlorella cell grows through the photosynthesis process with solar energy and carbon dioxide in fresh water. When it becomes 8 to 10 microns in size, division of its nucleus happens twice, where one parent cell divides into 4 cells daily.

Through Chlorella's energetic reproduction each cell increases to 4 cells every 20 to 24 hours. One Chlorella cell produces 4, second day 16, third day 64, etc. 10 thousand trillion cells weigh about 20 tons. No other plant grows as fast as Chlorella. Because of this, it has been studied extensively as a food for the future as our world population rapidly expands beyond the present day food production capacity of the earth.

Chlorella benefits us in 4 main ways:

1. Chlorella is a complete food providing nourishment directly at the cellular level

Chlorella is a very well-balanced package of essential nutrients. Along with its rich stores of complete protein, Chlorella also provides carbohydrates, essential fatty acids, minerals, vitamins, chlorophyll, fiber, antioxidants, RNA and DNA, its own unique Chlorella Growth Factor (CGF) and a wide variety of phytochemicals. The nutrients contained in Chlorella fulfills all the requirements for a superior health food. Working to maintain bodily health, prevent disease, and enhance recuperation, Chlorella can be thought of as a complete health supplement. It is truly the ultimate green food.

Chlorella works to directly nourish and stimulate each of the 60 trillion cells we have in our body. As cells are the fundamental building blocks of every part of our body, any restriction of their natural activities can lead to debilitating effects. Chlorella provides nutrients needed for these basic building blocks of our body - our cells.

Chlorella can help provide critical nutritional support that may be lacking in the diets of many people. It is an ideal supplement for the entire family, from infant to child to adult and seniors. It is also excellent for pets of all kinds.

Highly processed convenience foods have derailed our diets and health. Whole grains, legumes, fruits and vegetables have been substituted with nutrient-stripped carbohydrates such as processed flours and sugars. With today's depleted soils, growing methods, over-processing and lengthy shipping and storage times, even "healthy" natural foods often lack some of the key vitamins, nutrients and minerals our bodies need. Chlorella's nutritional support is excellent for people suffering from a lifetime of debilitating illness, or with broken down and weakened body systems.

2. Chlorella strengthens the immune system

If we want to help ourselves heal or even prevent disease, the key is to build up our immune system. Most viral infections and pathogenic intrusions can be successfully fought off if our cells are healthy and the metabolic pathways are clear.

Chlorella is a supreme booster of the immune system. This is one of the most significant benefits of this supplement. A strong, healthy immune system keeps pathogens in check and fends off illness.

Chlorella is well known in the Japanese scientific community as a "biological response modifier," which is a natural substance that improves the capacity of the body's immune system. Studies have consistently confirmed that Chlorella can provide critical benefits for the health of individuals with suppressed immune systems, especially when under stress.

3. Chlorella detoxifies and purifies the body

Detoxification refers to the removal of toxic substances from the body. This is a natural process the body is continually undergoing as we are exposed to these substances that may have entered from the outside - such as pesticide residues, use of pharmaceuticals or cigarettes, or are produced in the body such as in the colon due to inefficient metabolism in the body.

Chlorella works to clear the body of toxins, heavy metals and poisons. It can help our bodies to eliminate dioxins and other hormone disruptors.

Chlorella is our richest natural source of chlorophyll, which is a powerful cleanser and detoxifier, plus it's tough cell walls contain special fibers that bond to and remove numerous undesirables from our bodies. This helps relieve the burden of the liver and helps it to work more effectively.

4. Chlorella promotes healthy cellular growth and repair to slow down aging

All of the above aspects work together towards promoting longevity. These are what make Chlorella effective against the many problems resulting from debilitating modern lifestyles. All of these activities help us avoid illness and disease.

Chlorella also contains high levels of healing and anti-aging factors. Especially valuable are nucleic acids, RNA and DNA, and a specific compound unique to Chlorella, called Chlorella Growth Factor or CGF. This is what is responsible for Chlorella's high reproduction rate. In our bodies, this compound works to promote healthy cellular growth and repair. Our cells are continually renewing themselves. Given the proper nutritional support, with the encouragement of CGF and RNA and DNA, Chlorella not surprisingly has this important effect on us.

The healing effects in the body of these components of Chlorella are profound. Scientific studies demonstrate the potential Chlorella has to alleviate specific health problems such as high blood pressure, diabetes, malignant tumors, fibromyalgia and ulcers.

However, Chlorella is a God-created natural food, not a man-made drug or medication. Consuming Chlorella to heighten your immunity is fundamentally different from taking a drug to treat illness. Pharmaceutical medications are largely designed for symptom management. They are not designed to address the underlying problem causing the symptoms. Because the real problem remains, the symptoms will continue. Worse, consumption of strong medications means that over time, there will be side effects.

We all need to take an active role in caring for our own health. Consider ways to enhance your immunity to avoid getting sick rather than ways to reverse health problems when they present themselves.

Maintaining a proper and well-considered diet is key to effective preventive medicine. Common problems with most diets today include:

1. **We lack adequate fiber.**

2. **We consume too much sugar, refined carbohydrates and other processed foods.**

3. **We consume an excess of trans-fatty acids from processed fats (such as from fried foods, margarine, shortening and hydrogenated vegetable oils).**

4. **We consume inadequate Omega-3 essential fatty acids.**

5. **We lack many vitamins, mineral, phyto-chemicals and trace elements such as enzymes.**

Nutritional Value

Chlorella consists of approximately 60% protein in the form of amino acids. This is superior to other sources of protein from animals and vegetables which must be broken down to amino acids by the digestive enzymes in the stomach, and absorbed into the body through intestinal walls, before the body can utilize them for its own particular types of protein.

Among 22 different amino acids, all but 8 can be produced inside our body by using the other amino acids as material. These 8 amino acids can never be produced in our body, and must be consumed from food. These are called "essential amino acids". If any of these is even lacking, the others cannot function as well.

Chlorella contains 19 out of 22 different amino acids, and **all** 8 of the essential amino acids. Therefore, Chlorella is considered a complete protein.

CHLORELLA AMINO ACID CONTENT (%)

* **Essential Amino Acids**			
*Leucine	4.7	Glutamic Acid	5.8
*Valine	3.2	Aspartic Acid	4.7
*Lysine	3.1	Alanine	4.3
*Phenylalanine	2.8	Arginine	3.3
*Threonine	2.4	Glycine	3.1
*Isoleucine	2.3	Proline	2.5
*Methionine	1.3	Serine	2.0
*Tryptophan	0.5	Histidine	1.1
		Others	11.4

NUTRITIONAL PROFILE

Chlorella is a perfect food that provides nearly all of the body's nutritional needs. Levels shown are per 100 grams.

Beta Carotene . . . . 180 mg.
Biotin . . . . 1.91 mg.
Vitamin B-1 (Thiamine) . . . . 15 mg.
Vitamin B-2 (Riboflavin) . . . . 4.8 mg.
Vitamin B-3 (Niacin) . . . . 26 mg.
Vitamin B-5 (Pantothenic Acid) . . . . 13 mg.
Vitamin B-6 (Pyridoxine) . . . . .17 mg.
Vitamin B-12 . . . . 1.26 mg.
Vitamin C . . . . 15 mg.
Calcium . . . . 300 mg.
Chlorophyll . . . . .2,200 mg.
Copper . . . . 0.8 mg.
Vitamin E . . . . 09 mg.
Folic Acid . . . . 17 mg.
Iodine . . . . .60 mg.
Iron . . . . 108 mg.
Magnesium . . . . 399 mg.
Manganese . . . . 19.4 mg.
Phosphorus . . . . 1,000 mg.
Potassium . . . . .927 mg.
Selenium . . . . 7 mg.
Sodium . . . . 30 mg.
Zinc . . . . 70 mg.

Protein . . . . 60 %
Carbohydrates . . . . 20.1 %
Fiber . . . . 0.2 %
Fat . . . . 11 %
Unsaturated Fatty Acids (mostly Omega-3) 9.02 %
Saturated Fatty Acids . . . . 1.98 %

In addition, cultivating Chlorella makes good ecological sense since it produces 20 times as much protein as soybeans growing on an equal-sized area of land. Ounce for ounce Chlorella provides over twice the protein as soy, beef, or chicken and almost 20 times the protein as rice or potatoes.

PROTEIN COMPARISON (per 100 gm.)

Chlorella . . . . 60-67 %
Beef . . . . 24-27 %
Chicken . . . . 24 %
Fish . . . . 18-29 %
Eggs . . . . 13 %
Wheat . . . . 13 (incomplete) %
Rice . . . . 13 (incomplete) %
Potatoes . . . . 3 (incomplete) %

CGF - The Chlorella Powerhouse

A unique chemical complex to Chlorella protein called CGF (Chlorella Growth Factor) is believed to be the core of it's healing properties. All elements within Chlorella's nucleus (peptides, proteins, the nucleic acids (RNA and DNA), polysaccharides, beta glucans, sulfur and manganese combine to form CGF. It is found only in the nucleus of the cell.

In man, manganese is found in the highest concentrations in the bones, liver, pancreas and pituitary gland, which is the master gland of the endocrine system. Manganese deficiencies are associated with memory loss, aging, hormonal imbalances, metabolic disorders and much more, but manganese alone cannot explain all beneficial factors attributed to CGF.

Researchers have discovered that CGF is produced by Chlorella during the intense photosynthesis that enables Chlorella to grow so fast. Each cell multiplies into four new cells every 20-24 hours, and CGF promotes this rapid rate of reproduction.

This growth factor helps the growth of animals, microorganisms and renews our cells. Experiments with microorganisms, animals and children have shown that CGF promotes faster than normal growth without adverse side effects, and in adults, it appears to enhance RNA/DNA functions responsible for production of proteins, enzymes and energy at the cellular level, stimulating tissue repair and protecting cells against some toxic substances.

In children and adults CGF repairs damaged tissue and protects cells from toxins. CGF also helps promote the growth of beneficial bacteria in the colon.

CGF does not stimulate growth or weight gain in adults, nor is it known to stimulate the growth rate of any disease. It only stimulates growth in children and animals who have not yet reached their full, adult size. These results (increased selective growth and healing) cannot be explained by any other component in Chlorella other than its unique CGF. (Jenson)

Many scientists, scholars and doctors around the

world are presently trying to find out more about how CGF works. Some authorities report CGF is manufactured during the most intense periods of photosynthesis, incorporating the healing energy of sunlight within its structure. (Drucker)

Perhaps among the most interesting CGF research was done at a hospital where patients with long-standing wounds (gastric and peptic ulcers, and chronic gastritis) that refused to heal after treatment with standard medications. In these patients given liquid CGF in a matter of days, new tissue began to appear and all were soon healed completely. This clearly showed that CGF was capable of stimulating tissue repair when the body's healing sources were exhausted. (Jenson)

Dr. Bernard Jenson wrote in his book, *Chlorella: Gem of the Orient,* that CGF and the nucleic acids are the most valuable features of Chlorella because "*they lift the energy level of the body as a whole and because they repair and renew all organs, glands, and tissues of the body.*"

1. CGF helps maintain and repair cells

2. CGF increases energy levels

3. CGF stimulates growth of new cells

4. CGF supports immune function

The level of CGF in Chlorella supplements varies. While whole Chlorella typically contains about 5% CGF, liquid concentrates and powdered CGF extracts may contain 10-15 times this amount. Some special strains of Chlorella can exceed 20% CGF. The higher the level of CGF, the great the benefits.

Chlorella Offers Complete Nutrition

Chlorella is a complete storehouse of rich nutrients in addition to it's incredible protein content. It contains vitamins, minerals, carbohydrates, fiber, chlorophyll, enzymes, antioxidants and many other phytonutrients.

Chlorella provides vitamin A, Beta-carotene, vitamins B, C, E and K. Its minerals include calcium, iron, phosphorus, potassium, magnesium, zinc, manganese, sulfur, and several other trace minerals.

Chlorella is an especially rich source of lutein, a powerful antioxidant known to be highly beneficial for the eyes. Lutein is known to ward off vision problems such as cataracts, macular degeneration and retinal problems. Researchers at the Department of Nutritional Sciences at the University of Wisconsin demonstrated the importance of lutein in preventing the incidence of age-related nuclear cataracts in adults, 50-86 years of age. Lutein was the only carotenoid (out of five tested) demonstrating to protective against cataract development. (Lyle)

Some species of Chlorella (503 mg./100 mg.) contain 50 times more lutein than spinach (10.2 mg./100 mg. raw).

Chlorella's Health Benefits

Chlorella Detoxifies Your Body

Chlorella is a powerful detoxification aid for heavy metals and other pesticides. Numerous research projects in the U.S. and Europe indicate that Chlorella can also aid the body in breaking down persistent hydrocarbon and metallic toxins such as mercury, cadmium and lead, DDT and PCB while strengthening the immune system response. In Japan, interest in Chlorella has focused largely on its detoxifying properties - its ability to remove or neutralize poisonous substances from the body.

Chlorella is comprised of a fibrous, indigestible outer shell (20%) and its inner nutrients (80%). It is the fibrous material which has been proven to actually bind with the heavy metals, pesticides - such as PCBs, and other toxins - which can accumulate in our bodies, and remove them through the feces.

This cleansing of the blood, bowel and liver begins after Chlorella has been taken regularly for three months or more depending on the amount taken.

It is also this fibrous material in Chlorella which greatly augments healthy digestion and overall digestive tract health. Regular bowel movements is a very important aspect of our bodies natural cleansing process, but so many people are constipated. The longer this digestive waste remains in the body the more opportunity for the body actually reabsorb those same toxins that the body is trying to eliminate. If you eat two-three large meals daily, your bowels should move two-three times daily, anything less than this is an indication you are constipated. Most Americans are constipated because of a lack of dietary fiber in our highly processed diet. Fiber is what keeps things moving in the intestinal tract - and also attaches to heavy metals and other toxic debris and carries it out of the body.

Colon cancer is the second most common type of cancer today. We know that a refined, processed diet lacking fiber is the primary cause. In areas of the world where primitive diets are still consumed, such as rural Africa, colon cancer is non-existent.

The American Cancer Society recommends we consume 25-30 grams of fiber a day to prevent colon cancer and yet the average American only consumes 11 grams.

A clean bloodstream, with an abundance of red blood cells to carry oxygen, is necessary to a strong natural defense system. Chlorella's cleansing action on the bowel and other elimination channels, as well as its protection of the liver, helps keep the blood clean. Clean blood insures that metabolic wastes are efficiently carried away from the tissues. The process of detoxification in the body is normal and crucial for the overall health of all the systems of the body. Because Chlorella aids in this process, immunity can be enhanced and all systems can work more efficiently.

Dr. Ichimura at the Toyama University gave 30 tablets (6 grams) of Chlorella daily to 30 patients suffering from heavy metal toxicity. He reported that heavy metals were discharged in intestinal movements. Today, environmental contamination is often caused by chemical heavy metals and this report on Chlorella is considered as a remarkable research finding. (Hagino, Ichimura)

Chlorophyll is a key detoxifier

Chlorella gets its name from the high amount of chlorophyll it possesses. Chlorella contains more chlorophyll per gram than any other plant. Chlorophyll is one of the greatest food substances for cleansing the bowel and other elimination systems, such as the liver and the blood.

Green algae are the highest sources of chlorophyll in the plant world. And of all the green algae studied so far, Chlorella has the highest, often ranging from 2 to 5% pure natural chlorophyll. Chlorella contains up to five times more chlorophyll than wheat grass, up to ten times more than spirulina, up to 12 times more than barley, and up to 50 times more than Alfalfa (depending on species and grade).

Chlorella is richer in chlorophyll, beta carotene and lutein than most green and yellow vegetables. These natural pigments are absorbed through the digestive tract, and therefore they can be fully expected to be effective.

CHLOROPHYLL

Chlorophyll, the green pigment in plants that helps plant cells capture and convert sunlight into energy, is believed to be very beneficial to humans. Anecdotal and popular use of foods containing chlorophyll shows it helps cleanse the bloodstream, deodorize bad breath and body odor, deactivate carcinogenic substances and halt tooth decay. In addition, inflammatory conditions such as arthritis and stomach ulcers respond well to algae supplementation, writes Paul Pitchford, author of *Healing with Whole Foods* (North Atlantic Books). Chlorophyll may also help decrease cellular damage caused by environmental carcinogens by acting as an antioxidant, writes chemist Karl J. Abrams in his book, *Algae to the Rescue!* (Logan House).

Pitchford and others theorize that chlorophyll mimics human hemoglobin. "The ability of chlorophyll to enrich the blood and treat anemia may be due to a similarity in molecular structure between hemoglobin (red blood cells) and chlorophyll," he writes. "Their molecules are virtually identical except for their central atom: The center of the chlorophyll molecule is magnesium, whereas iron occupies the central position in hemoglobin."

Chlorophyll help detoxify the body because it absorbs and inactivates toxic materials.

Hemoglobin is the protein in our red blood cells which binds with oxygen and gives blood its bright red color. Chlorophyll cells are nearly identical to hemoglobin, with one exception: Chlorophyll has a magnesium molecule at its center while hemoglobin has an iron molecule at the center of it. This is important because magnesium is essential for the heart to function properly. Every time our heart beats, it requires magnesium to do so.

Molecular Structure Comparison of Red Blood Cell and Chlorophyll

Chlorophyll is also effective against anemia and stimulates the production of red blood cells in the body. Several researchers have suggested the use of chlorophyll as a medical therapy for anemia. It also helps carry oxygen around the body and to the brain. For this reason, Chlorella is sometimes called a 'Brain Food'.

Effects of Chlorella chlorophyll pigments:
1. Antimutagenic: *against Aflatoxin B (mold),*
   Benzo (a) pyren (tobacco),
   Heterocyclic amin (burnt foods)
2. Protects stomach walls inhibiting pepsin activity
3. Deodorizer (body odor, bad breath, etc.)
4. Anti-oxidant
5. Excretes toxic dioxin chemicals

Effects of Chlorella beta-carotene pigments:

Provitamin A, an essential fat-soluble micro-
  nutrient
Antioxidant
Prevention of arteriosclerosis
Anti-cancer

Effect of Chlorella lutein pigments:

Antioxidant - specifically prevents lipid-
  preoxidation that occurs in blood plasma and
  eyes. Lutein is the most effective carotenoid for
  this action.

Pigment Content Comparison in Green & Yellow Vegetables

Vegetable (10 grams)	Chlorophyll	Beta-carotene	Lutein
Broccoli	120 mg	.7 mg	2 mg.
Cabbage	60 mg.	.08 mg.	.3 mg.
Carrots	trace	7-17 mg.	.3 mg.
Spinach	130 mg.	14 mg.	15 mg.
Chlorella*	3,700 mg.	106 mg.	503 mg.

* - Levels of various species of Chlorella may vary slightly

Chlorella Improves Digestion

Chlorella contains several components helpful for our digestive system; enzymes, fiber and its high chlorophyll content is given the credit for helping people eliminate chronic bad breath in just a few days on Chlorella. Foul smelling stools are also greatly improved as digestion is improved and toxins are eliminated.

Chlorella contains natural digestive and other enzymes. Chlorella also causes the friendly lactic bacteria in the gut to multiply at four times the usual rate, improving digestion and the absorption of nutrients into the bloodstream. This bacteria also helps combat the overproduction of pathogens common to the intestinal tract such as candida albicans (also referred to as a yeast infection). The B vitamins in Chlorella also aid in this important process.

The indigestible Chlorella cell wall acts as a fiber in the bowels, stimulating peristalsis. It also strengthens the intestine and relieves chronic constipation.

Chlorella contains enzymes such as chlorophyllase and pepsin, which are two digestive enzymes which perform a number of important functions in the body. Chlorella has many different types of enzymes that our bodies need.

Chlorella Helps Balance Your pH

pH is a reference to the state of alkalinity or acidity in the body. 7 is neutral - neither acidic or alkaline. Below 7 is acidic, increasing in acidity as the number decreases, above 7 is alkaline, increasing in alkalinity as the number increases.

It's important that we maintain a proper pH of the body fluids, which is ideally about 7.4 (slightly alkaline). However, because of our poor diet of junk food, overcooked, processed foods, fast food, which includes soft drinks (pH of 2.7), most of us are not balanced and are too acidic.

pH of the body can be tested with either saliva or urine. Urine is believed to be more accurate as saliva can be easily altered with food, or other things in the mouth. If you are testing saliva, do not have anything in your mouth for 30 minutes prior to testing or the results will not be accurate.

An environment in the body which is too acidic:

1. Creates an ideal opportunity for pathogens (bacteria, viruses and fungus) to survive.

2. Reduces the level of oxygen creating an ideal opportunity for cancer cells to thrive.

3. Can create tissue damage in our arteries which cholesterol sticks to creating plaque build-up. This can result in clogging of the arteries (heart disease and stroke).

Popular Foods That Contribute to an Acidic System

Acid-forming foods should make up only 20% of our diet. Here is a brief list of items which lower our pH (making it more acidic). **Reduce your intake of these foods.**

Coffee, soft drinks, alcoholic drinks, cocoa
Sugar and most sweeteners and deserts
Animal fat, butter, cream, cheese, milk (store),
    Meat, seafood, poultry, egg whites
Processed oils, margarine, crisco
Black and green tea
All grains and grain products (**EXCEPT** oats,
    buckwheat, amaranth, quinoa, millet)
Flour products, pasta
Beans, lentils
Most nuts (**EXCEPT** coconut and almonds)
Condiments and dressings
Pharmaceuticals
Tobacco

Increase your consumption of alkaline-forming foods. These include:
Chlorella
Almost all vegetables, especially green
Most fruit - Grapefruit, oranges, lemons,
    pineapple, berries, sour apples, sour
    grapes, sour plums
Potatoes (esp. the skin), pumpkin, squash
Soybeans
Yams, sweet potatoes
Acidophilus milk, buttermilk, yogurt
Milk (raw only -- human, cow or goat)

Maintaining proper pH of the body is very important because most diseases start, live and thrive in an acidic environment and do not live well in an alkaline environment. Cancer rates have risen steadily so that authorities predict one-third of all people in the U. S. will get cancer in their lifetime.

The rise of fast, junk and processed foods match those of rising cancer rates. Including whole foods like Chlorella in your diet is one step toward improving your odds against developing cancer in the future.

Chlorella is rich in minerals which the body uses to buffer an acidic system. Most diets today are mineral deficient and is probably the main reason so many people suffer from health problems associated with an acidic system.

Processing and refining of foods, decreases the mineral content and therefore increases the acidic effect it has on our bodies. Eat natural, unrefined foods as much as possible!

Chlorella Normalizes Blood Sugar and Blood Pressure

Studies have shown that Chlorella tends to normalize blood sugar in cases of hypoglycemia. In hypoglycemia, blood sugar is too low. Proper levels of blood sugar are necessary for normal brain function, heart function and energy metabolism, all of which are crucial in sustaining good health and preventing disease.

High blood pressure is one of the major risk factors in heart attack and stroke, which account for more fatalities in the United States than any other disease. Laboratory experiments have shown that regular use of Chlorella reduces high blood pressure and prevents strokes. (Merchant)

Chlorella Benefits Ulcerative Colitis, Fibromyalgia and other Chronic Health Problems

Researchers at Virginia Commonwealth University, Medical College of Virginia, Richmond, found promising results using Chlorella to treat chronic health problems such as ulcerative colitis and fibromyalgia. They demonstrated the potential of Chlorella to relieve symptoms, improve quality of life, and normalize body functions in patients with fibromyalgia or ulcerative colitis. The effects may be attributable to enhanced overall immune function. (Merchant)

Animal studies have also shown Chlorella's protective effect against stress-induced peptic ulcers. It is believed to prevent ulcer formation mainly through the "immune-brain-gut" axis and protection of the gastric mucosa. (Tanaka)

Chronic Fatigue Syndrome (CFS) - Prolonged fatigue, fever, joint pain, and depression are the common symptoms of this chronic condition. Support to the immune system and adrenal glands is recognized as the most effective treatment. The adrenal glands can be nourished with vitamins C, B complex and zinc - all of which are provided in Chlorella. Many people report great benefit taking Chlorella against CFS with improved energy and reduced symptoms.

Note: CoQ10 (about 300 mg. daily) is also recommended.

Chlorella Has Anti-Aging Effects

Not only does it contain powerful antioxidants, Chlorella has an abundance of nucleic acids, RNA (ribonucleic acid) and DNA (deoxyribonucleic acid), found primarily in the CGF. RNA and DNA is the reproductive (genetic) substance found in every cell which rejuvenates cellular activity. It is often referred to as the "essence of life" which retards the aging process.

Dr. Benjamin Frank, author of *Doctor Frank's No-Aging Diet,* suggests that human RNA/DNA production slows down progressively as people age, resulting in lower levels of vitality and increased vulnerability to various diseases. He recommends a diet rich in nucleic acids to counter this "aging" process. Chlorella is the richest food source of nucleic acids containing 3% RNA and 0.3% DNA.

When our RNA and DNA are in good repair and able to function most efficiently, our bodies are able to use nutrients more effectively, get rid of toxins and avoid disease. Cells are able to repair themselves and the energy level and vitality of the whole body is raised. The breakdown of DNA and RNA in the cells is believed to be one of the main factors in aging and degenerative diseases. (Frank)

Nucleic acids in digestion and assimilation are broken down and combined with other nutrients such as vitamin B-12, peptides and polysaccharides. That means that the DNA and RNA we eat do not directly replace human cellular DNA and RNA, but their amino acid combinations after digestion and assimilation immediately provide the "building blocks" for repair of our genetic material.

As people age, cellular processes slow down. The cell wall, which regulates fluids, intake of nutrients and expulsion of wastes, becomes less functional. Nutrient intake is less efficient and more toxic waste remains in the cells.

This leads to an increasing acidic condition in the body that favors many kinds of chronic and degenerative diseases. When we have a sufficient intake of foods rich in DNA and RNA to protect our own cellular nucleic acids, the cell wall continues to function efficiently, keeping the cell clean and well nourished.

There is great potential benefits from using Chlorella regularly. The RNA and DNA in Chlorella are invaluable to aid cellular repair and restoration. Chlorella protects our health by supporting vital cellular-level functions that keep bodies fit.

Brewer's yeast is known to be a good source of RNA, but sardines contain 10 times more than Brewer's yeast (343 mg. per 100 grams). Chlorella actually provides 10 times more RNA than sardines with 3,000 mg. per 100 grams!

Dr. Jenson wrote in his book, *Chlorella: Gem of the Orient.*

> *"In my travels around the world, searching for the secrets of long life, I found out that the foods people eat have a great deal to do with youthfulness, the repair and rebuilding of tissue, and a long healthy life. When I visited Charlie Smith in Bartow, Florida, he was 135 years old, healthy, clear minded and with a wonderful memory. It nearly blew my mind when I found out he had been living the last 30 years on canned sardines and crackers!"*

Chlorella Benefits the Immune System

Chlorella supports the entire body which results in an overall strengthening of the immune system. A system less burdened by toxins and debris can work more effectively and every aspect of our health benefits. The complete nutritional support provided by Chlorella also indirectly supports the immune system. Disease preys on an undernourished body.

Chlorella also directly of certain aspects of the immune system by inducing higher levels of interferon (a natural anti-cancer and anti-viral agent in the body) and stimulates the activity of tumor necrosis factor, T-cells, macrophages (cells that actively protect against disease by digesting foreign substances in the body). This enhances the immune system's ability to combat bacteria, viruses, chemicals and foreign proteins. (Pugh, Hasegawa)

Chlorella Growth Factor (CGF) also aids immunity as it stimulates healing and replacement of cellular tissue.

In addition to support of the immune system nutritionally, Chlorella contains specific nutrients such as beta-carotene (known to destroy cancer cells), and antioxidant vitamins C and E and selenium. Beta carotene, lutein and zinc are also a few of the numerous antioxidants provided by Chlorella.

Health Applications of Chlorella

Alzheimer's - The use of aluminum in deodorants and cooking utensils has been associated with an increase risk for Alzheimer's disease. Regular long term use of Chlorella cleanses the system from such heavy metals. A greater supply of oxygen to the brain aids alertness and mental focus in Alzheimer's' patients and those suffering from dementia and also Attention Deficit Disorder (ADD).

Anemia - Chlorella's rich stores of chlorophyll stimulate the production of red blood cells and is effective against anemia.

The blood-building vitamin B-12 is found in Chlorella among the highest concentrations of any food. Chlorella may serve an an excellent B-12 source for vegetarians as few non-animal sources of B-12 are available.

Chlorella's fiber and chlorophyll content also promotes healthy intestinal bacterial production which also produces vitamin B-12.

Antiinflammatory - Studies at the Department of Pathology, Oklahoma State University Center for Health Sciences, examined the prevalence of an antiinflammatory activity in Chlorella and selected algae.

They found the inhibition of histamine release from mast cells. Mast cells are responsible for the inflammatory response and histamine release in the body. Antihistamines are commonly used for allergy and cold symptoms but they are not without side effects. Chlorella may be a natural, non-toxic alternative without side effects. (Price)

Arthritis - Because of the high mineral content in Chlorella, it is very alkaline and can help to neutralize the body's pH. Our pH levels are frequently too acidic as a result of consuming too many processed foods and carbonated soft drinks. Arthritis is one (of many) conditions associated with an acidic constitution.

Chlorella also contains vitamins A, C and E and selenium, which together combat arthritis. Chlorella's outer wall contains glucosamine, which is very important for health of cartilage, tendons, ligaments and other connective tissue.

Cancer - Chlorella contains numerous components that support the immune system, our built-in defense mechanism against cancerous cells. The body was designed with the ability to search out and destroy abnormal cells in the body which could be potentially cancerous. If this ability of our white blood cells (macrophages and T-cells) is weakened due to lack of nutritional support or overwork due to high levels of free radicals, toxins or other debris, our risk of cancer increases.

Animal studies show that components in Chlorella demonstrate anti-cancer immunity through T cell activation in lymphoid organs and enhances recruitment of these cells to the tumor sites. (Tanaka, Noda, Justo)

Chlorella vulgaris was fed a daily diet with 10% dried powder of Chlorella to tumor-bearing mice. In the mice given Chlorella, the growth of tumors was significantly suppressed in an antigen-specific manner mediated by cytostatic T cells. (Tanaka)

Japanese researchers found that a glycoprotein prepared from Chlorella vulgaris is a biological response modifier (BRM) which exhibits protective activities against tumor growth and immunosuppression. (Hasegawa)

Candida Albicans - Chlorella helps control candida yeast overgrowth by helping maintain an alkaline system and by encouraging healthy bacterial growth in the intestinal tract through its fibrous cellular wall.

Also suggested to control yeast is to eliminate all sugar and refined foods. These feed the yeast, create an acidic system and encourage their proliferation.

Cardiovascular Health - Chlorella, the richest natural source of chlorophyll, has a structure almost identical to that of haemoglobin. Chlorophyll cells have a magnesium molecule at the center, Hemoglobin has iron in the center. Magnesium is essential for heart health and is also known to be beneficial against high blood pressure.

Chlorella also provides Omega-3 fatty acids, which are known to protect against heart disease. Research programs have indicated that regular use of Chlorella helps guard against heart disease, reduce high blood pressure and lower blood cholesterol levels. (Merchant)

Animals fed a high cholesterol diet for 10 weeks remarkably increased their serum total cholesterol and the beta-lipoprotein cholesterol levels which are associated with aortic lesions where plague accumulates. Among those given Chlorella, the increase of total and beta-lipoprotein cholesterol level was suppressed and the development of aortic lesions was significantly inhibited. (Sano)

Circulation - Chlorella is a biological response modifier (BRM) which helps the body deal with stress. Stress releases hormones such as cortisol which have a negative effect upon circulation and many other aspects in the body.

Japanese researchers showed that oral administration of Chlorella significantly suppressed the increase in serum corticosterone level in psychologically stressed mice. This suggest that Chlorella prevents psychological stress and maintain homeostasis in the face of external environmental changes. (Hasegawa)

Chlorella helps normalize the flow of fluids through

the body. About 15% of the fluid in our body is blood, the lymph systems carries another 70%. Blood is moved through the body's circulatory system by the heart "pump," while nearly 500 nodes filter lymph fluid as it circulates throughout the body. Both systems are fundamental to our health. If the flow of these fluids through the body is restricted, the body's ability to function properly is affected and we become suscepti- ble to debilitating effects.

Common symptoms include a feeling of heaviness in the arms or difficulty turning the head. These are often due to a problem with obstructed flow of lymph fluids. The superior nutritional balance afforded by Chlorella helps ease and normalize the flow of the essential liquids in our metabolic pathways.

Specifically, Chlorella counters many of the effects of poor adult health due to sedentary life styles or poor nutrition. These effects arise from problems with the flow of fluids through our metabolic pathways such as blood or lymph, so clearing the pathways can help pre- vent problems arising from poor health practices.

Liver Disease - The liver is the detoxifying organ in the body. It removes chemical food additives, bacterial wastes, incompletely digested protein, pesticides, heavy metals, toxins formed in the bowel, and in some people drugs (including prescription) and alcohol. An over- worked liver will become sluggish and eventually allow poisons to infiltrate the bloodstream. This affects the health of every organ and gland in the body, including the liver.

Chlorella primarily aids the liver as it greatly relieves the burden of the liver by removing toxins from the body.

Chlorophyll cleanses and stimulates the bowels and builds up the hemoglobin level in the blood. Enhanced bowel health improves removal of cholesterol, fat and other toxic waste. The RNA/DNA is believed to stimulate liver tissue repair at the cellular level. The liver has the highest level of regeneration power of all organs in the body.

In Germany, Dr. Herman Fink showed the benefit of green algae on the liver. Rats fed a diet of skim milk all died of liver disease. Almost all the rats fed a diet of egg whites also died of liver disease. Rats fed a diet of green algae remained healthy. (Steenblock)

Excess alcohol leads to cirrhosis, a potentially fatal disease, where scar tissue blocks veins and causes organ failure.

There are numerous reports of reversal of cirrhosis of the liver using high levels of Chlorella (6 grams daily plus CGF liquid) after 3 or 4 months. (Jenson)

Pets - Ever wondered why pets love to eat grass? They have nutritional needs that give them cravings just like us! What does grass contain? It is rich in minerals and chlorophyll!

Pets love Chlorella and it is so good for them! The following health problems are reported to have benefited from giving their pet Chlorella:

In cats: Pulling fur out, house plant eating (many of which are poisonous).

In dogs: Hot spots (itching), suppressed immunity, thinning coat, allergies, arthritis, improved eyes and enhanced energy.

There are several companies that manufacture Chlorella wafers just for pets. They will eat what they know is good for them! My dog loves raw broccoli, carrots, actually most fruit and vegetables and Chlorella too!

Wound healing - The high amount of chlorophyll accelerates wound and burn healing when applied topically. Chlorella also promotes the healing of diabetic skin ulcers, which can lead to amputation if they become infected. This is thought to be due to an increased production of TNF (Tumor Necrosis Factor) which promotes fibroblasts, cells the body uses to repair wounds. Taking Chlorella on a regular basis over a long period of time will increase the body's ability to heal itself of cuts, scrapes, rashes and more serious wounds without the need to apply it externally. (Merchant)

Safety & Side Effects

Chlorella can safely be taken by adults, the elderly children and infants. In fact, Chlorella in pure water is recommended for infants who do not have access to mother's milk or who are allergic to formula or cow's milk. This is actually superior to most formulas or cow's milk which do not supply essential fatty acids which are crucial for optimal development of the immune system, vision and brain.

As whole food, rather than a concentrated extract Chlorella can be taken in large amounts with no unpleasant side effects. Chlorella has not been found to have a single detrimental affect on human health. It is almost impossible to take too much Chlorella.

Because of Chlorella's natural ability to remove toxins from our cells and tissues, the following initial reactions may occur in individuals with a high level of intestinal toxic build-up:

1. Intestinal gases may be released due to the rejuvenation of the action of the intestines. This will cease as the intestines are cleansed.

2. Nausea and slight fever may occur in a small number of people for 2-3 days. These reactions are most prevalent in those who need Chlorella's cleansing the most.

3. Because the skin is also an excretory organ of cleansing, some individuals may initially experience acne, pimples, rashes, boils or eczema. This is a sign of the body's attempts to regain internal balance as it actively works to expel toxins.

How To Use Chlorella

For general health maintenance, a daily dose of 2-3 grams is recommended. If it is being taken to relieve specific symptoms, the dosage should be doubled to 4-6 grams. Athletes and individuals who push their bodies to the limit may take 10 grams or more daily; with Chlorella, more IS better!

Since Chlorella is a whole food it can be taken anytime, with or without food. However, to take advantage of its benefits for the digestive system, it is best taken just before meals.

Chlorella is available in tablet, capsule and powder form. Liquid CGF concentrate (from Chlorella), which is about 10-15 times higher in CGF than whole Chlorella is also available, but it is quite expensive in this form.

To use Chlorella powder: Add 1-2 teaspoons of Chlorella powder to water, juice, yogurt or smoothie and stir well. One level teaspoon contains approximately 2-3 grams.

In Japan, because of it's high content of minerals and other useful nutrients such as CGF, Chlorella powder is often added to many foods such as soup, baked goods, fruit juice, noodles, honey, syrup, tea. etc.

Chlorella is excellent for use during fasting as it provides complete nutrition and also aids in the detoxification process.

How To Select Your Chlorella

1. Look for high levels of the following key marker components in Chlorella (listed in order of importance): Chlorella Growth Factor (CGF), Chlorophyll and Protein. Typical value guidelines are:

Marker	Poor	Average	Excellent
CGF	< 5%	10%	>15%
Chlorophyll	<1.5%	2.5%	> 3.5%
Protein	< 50%	55%	> 60%

Different brands of Chlorella offer different sub-strains, growing conditions and procedures which can greatly affect the potency of Chlorella. For example, some brands can be several times higher in CGF and chlorophyll than other brands due to selective breeding, superior cultivation techniques and quality control practices.

2. Ensure Chlorella's tough cell wall is broken or cracked to improve digestibility as whole Chlorella is less than 50% digestible. Traditionally, Chlorella's cell walls have been broken by heat, chemical processing or milling. Milling grinds up the Chlorella to increase digestibility but this process also exposes the nutrients within the cell wall to increased oxidation and can reduce potency and shelf stability.

Today, high pressure jet-spray drying is the pre-ferred means of cell wall breakdown as it typically achieves over 80% digestibility without compromising potency or shelf life.

3. Choose a brand of Chlorella that is grown out-doors in clean, mineral-rich water with lots of natural sunlight. Japan's subtropical climate is perfect for the outdoor growing of Chlorella. Chlorella grown indoors in cement tanks have significantly lower concentrations of all the key marker components listed above plus lower levels of vitamins and minerals, especially calci-um and iron. Natural sunlight can not be reproduced by any man made device.

4. Choose brands from the undisputed leader in Chlorella development and cultivation. Japan is by far the world's largest and most experienced Chlorella producer.

5. Choose brands of tablets and capsules that con-tain no binders or fillers or powders which are 100% Chlorella.

Commonly Asked Q's & A's

Q: What is Chlorella used for?

A: It can be used as a nutrient-dense whole food or a food supplement taken to ensure you are obtaining all of your dietary needs. Fatigue and mental depression, which are so common today, are signals from the body that something is wrong. Chlorella serves as an overall health and immune booster to encourage and maintain good health.

Q: How long does one need to take it to see results?

A: Keep in mind that Chlorella is a food and not a drug. While some people see effects in just a few days, 2-3 months may be needed to realize the full effect of its many benefits. Once the body has less toxic load the organs and glands can begin restoration towards optimal functioning. This can take even longer to realize the full benefit of this. Thus, it can take even longer to realize all the benefits of taking Chlorella.

Q: What is the difference between Chlorella and Spirulina or blue-green algae?

A: Spirulina and blue-green algae are actually not algae but cyanobacteria. Both are high in protein and vitamins but they lack the cell nucleus that characterizes Chlorella as a complete unicellular organism. Spirulina is cultivated like Chlorella but blue green algae grows wild in lakes and waterways, consuming whatever nutrients are in the water. Some species of cyanobacteria are toxic just like mushrooms and some land plants. Companies that harvest wild species of blue-green algae from natural lakes cannot have the same degree of control as growing chlorella and harvesting wild algae presents a far greater risk of contamination by cyanobacterial toxins. Chlorella contains up to 10 times more chlorophyll than spirulina and up to 20 times more than blue green algae, making it a much superior detoxifier. Chlorella is also a more complete and higher quality source of protein and of course Chlorella is the only source of CGF which is responsible for many of its healing and anti-aging properties.

Q: Is Chlorella good for vegetarians?

A: It is excellent for vegetarians due to it's B-12 content and wide range of amino acids, including all 8 essentials. These nutrients can sometimes be deficient in non-meat eaters.

Q: Is Chlorella good for athletes and body-builders?

A: Athletes tend to push themselves physically to the limit. This creates a great stress if proper nutrition is not there to support those demands. The high level of a wide range of amino acids ensures optimal healing and recovery to muscle tissue, joints and any other area of the body. Thus, plus Chlorella's overall nutritional food value, high levels of nucleic acids and CGF makes it a fantastic food supplement for all athletes.

Q: What is the best way to ensure digestibility with Chlorella's tough outer wall?

A: Every manufacturer of Chlorella claims to have a special cell wall treatment to improve digestion. Most advanced producers today use super high pressure jet spray drying which creates deep cracks in the cell walls, making the nutrients within available to us, but keeps them contained and intact within the cell walls until they are actually consumed. Others actually mill the Chlorella which grinds and collapses the entire Chlorella cell into very small fragments, therefore exposing the nutrients contained within Chlorella, reducing shelf life and requiring significantly more extensive packaging. Both methods are effective and offer 80% or higher digestibility. Don't be mislead by special patented procedures that claim only their process increases digestibility.

Q: Can Chlorella be used topically?

A: Yes. Chlorella powder can be mixed with water into a thick paste and applied over cuts, scrapes, rashes or wounds to help facilitate healing.

The CGF makes it an effective healer of human tissue. After consuming Chlorella for approximately one year, you should notice significant improvement in the healing of cuts, scrapes, and wounds without the need to apply it topically.

Q: Are there any side effects or interactions with other supplements or drugs using Chlorella?

A: None have been reported. It is very safe.

Q: *How does Chlorella taste?*

A: It tastes GREEN! Try adding Chlorella powder to fruit smoothies or juices such as apple, white grape, pineapple or orange. The natural sugars in these combine well with Chlorella.

Q: *Is it true that Chlorella can help with weight loss?*

A: This has been one of the reported benefits by Chlorella users. Many people report that taking Chlorella before meals acts like an appetite suppressant. Because it contains such a wide variety of nutrients and fiber, Chlorella can easily satisfy our nutritional needs and therefore, our appetite is diminished.

Many times we eat to satisfy a biological craving the body has, but instead of eating the correct food, we eat processed refined foods lacking the very nutrients the body is craving. Because the fiber is removed in refined foods, they do not fill us up and we end up eating more calories than we realize. This easily leads to weight gain or makes it much more difficult for us to lose weight. Chlorella is very low calorie, but nutrient dense food to satisfy those nutritional needs to cease those cravings. Chlorella's valuable fiber also helps us feel more full.

Also Chlorella is known to be an adaptogen or a biological response modifier (BRM) meaning it helps the body lower hormones associated with stress. These stress hormones have numerous negative effects on the body that can cause us to eat more, but our ability to digest that food slows down, leading to weight gain. If we lower those stress hormones (as with Chlorella) our food cravings diminish and our digestive system can work more effectively!

Q: What other health benefits are associated with Chlorella?

A: Chlorella is mostly recognized for it's rich composition of phytochemicals that support the body's natural self-defense mechanism, detoxify and nourish the body and assist in achieving longevity and well-being.

It makes sense that if your body is weary, run down, undernourished and etc. that where ever there is a weak area in the body, that area will probably suffer and with the proper nutritional support those problems can be reversed. Chlorella is not some miracle cure. The human body is the miracle as it was created to heal itself if given the proper nutritional support to do so.

Many different health benefits have been reported by individuals using Chlorella. The following is a list of reported benefits, even though many of them have not been scientifically investigated, they do physiologically make sense if one considers all of the nutrients provided in Chlorella, the detoxification effects, the anti-aging effects, and on and on.

Increase energy and stamina
Aid stomach/duodenal ulcers
Eliminate constipation
Reduce chronic fatigue
Reduce fibromyalgia
Reduce neuralgia
Healthy weight gain
Reduce allergic reactions
Lower blood pressure
Help control diabetes
Help control blood sugar
Support immune function
Reduce rheumatism

Improve chronic conditions
Promote an alkaline system
Regulate appetite
Reduce food cravings
Reduce colds and flu
Reduce candida overgrowth
Improve circulation disorders
Aid skin problems/rashes
Lower cholesterol
Improve sleep
Decrease pain
Aid fertility problems
Aid hair loss
Reduce headaches
Reduce diarrhea
Sharpen memory
Heal athlete's foot
Aid in wound repair
Detoxify the body
Reduce heavy metals
Remove fat
Reduce stiffness
Prevent hangovers
Menstrual disorders
Aid internal bleeding
Eliminate halitosis
Heal hemorrhoids
Benefit liver disorders
Promote longevity

Chlorella contains all the components essential to life, making it the most nutritionally potent whole food available!

References

Abrams, K.; *Algae to the Rescue!* (Logan House), 1997.

Barrett JR.; Cancer. Plants provide prevention. Environ Health Perspect. 2002 Apr;110(4):A180.

Dantas DC, Kaneno R, Queiroz ML.; The effects of Chlorella vulgaris in the protection of mice infected with Listeria monocytogenes. Role of natural killer cells. Immunopharmacol Immunotoxicol. 1999 Aug;21(3):609-19.

Fortune JM, Dickey JS, Lavrukhin OV, Van Etten JL, Lloyd RS, Osheroff N.; Site-specific DNA cleavage by Chlorella virus topoisomerase II. Biochemistry. 2002 Oct 1;41(39):11761-9.

Frank, B.; Doctor Frank's No Aging Diet, Doubleday, 1976.

Hagino N, Ichimura S.; Effect of Chlorella on fecal and urinary cadmium excretion in "Itai-itai" disease. Nippon Eiseigaku Zasshi. 1975 Apr;30(1):77.

Hasegawa T, Kimura Y, Hiromatsu K, Kobayashi N,; Effect of hot water extract of Chlorella vulgaris on cytokine expression patterns in mice with murine acquired immunodeficiency syndrome after infection with Listeria monocytogenes. Immunopharmacology. 1997 Jan;35(3):273-82.

Hasegawa T, Noda K, Kumamoto S.; Chlorella vulgaris culture supernatant (CVS) reduces psychological stress-induced apoptosis in thymocytes of mice. Int J Immunopharmacol. 2000 Nov;22(11):877-85.

Harada H, Noro T, Kamei Y.; Selective antitumor activity in vitro from marine algae from Japan coasts. Biol Pharm Bull. 1997 May;20(5):541-6.

Hasegawa T, Ito K, Ueno S, Kumamoto S, Ando Y,.; Oral administration of hot water extracts of Chlorella vulgaris reduces IgE production against milk casein in mice. Int J Immunopharmacol. 1999 May;21(5):311-23.

Hasegawa T, Matsuguchi T, Noda K, Tanaka K, Kumamoto S, Shoyama Y, Yoshikai Y. Toll-like receptor 2 is at least partly involved in the antitumor activity of glycoprotein from Chlorella vulgaris. Int Immunopharmacol. 2002 Mar;2(4):579-89.

Hasegawa T, Noda K, Kumamoto S,; Chlorella vulgaris culture supernatant (CVS) reduces psychological stress-induced apoptosis in thymocytes of mice. Int J Immunopharmacol. 2000 Nov;22(11):877-85.

Ichimura S. Effect of Chlorella on skin cancer of Black Foot patients in south Formosa, Nippon Eiseigaku Zasshi. 1975 Apr;30(1):66.
Jenson, B.: Chlorella: Gem of The Orient, 1987, Escondido, Ca.

Justo GZ, Silva MR, Queiroz ML.; Effects of the green algae Chlorella vulgaris on the response of the host hematopoietic system to intraperitoneal ehrlich ascites tumor transplantation in mice. Immunopharmacol Immunotoxicol. 2001 Feb;23(1):119-32.

Kanazawa Medical College Dept. of Serology: Effects of various preparations made from Chlorella Pyrenoidosa cells on the defense mechanism (immune resistance). Scient. Rep. on Chlorella in Japan. 66-70, 1980. Silpaque Publishing, Japan.

Kirschmann, J.; Nutrition Almanac, Bismark, ND, 2001.

Konishi, F.; Tanaka, K.; Himeno, K.; et al: Anti-tumor effect induced by a hot water extract of Chlorella vulgaris. Resistance to Meth-A tumor growth mediated by CE-induced polymorphonuclear leucocytes. Cancer Immunology and Immunotherapy; 19, 73-78, 1985.
Koniyama, K.; Hirok awa, Y.; Mocota, T.; et al: An acidic polysaccharide,

Chion A, from Chlorella Pyrenoidosa. Anti-tumor activity and immunological response. Chemotherapy, 34, 302-307, 1986.

Kuniaki, T.; Yoshifumi, T.; Tsuruta, M.; et al: Oral administration of Chlorella vulgaris augments concomitant anti-tumor immunity. Immunopharmacology and Immunotoxicology, 12 (2), 277-291, 1990.

Leng-Fang, W., et al.: Protective Effect of Chlorella on the Hepatic Damage Induced by Ethionine in Rats. J. Formosan Medical Assoc. Vol. 78, No. 12, (Dec. 1979), pp 1010-1019.

Lin, J.K., et al.: Effect of Chlorella on Serum Cholesterol of Rats. Taiwan Medical Science Journal, Sept. 1981.

Lyle BJ; Mares-Perlman JA; Klein BE; Klein R; Palta M; Bowen PE; Greger JL; Serum carotenoids and tocopherols and incidence of age-related nuclear cataract. Department of Nutritional Sciences, University of Wisconsin, Madison. Am J Clin Nutr 1999 Feb;69(2):272-7.

Matsueda S., Ichita, J.: Studies on Antitumor Active Glycoprotein From Chlorella vulgaris. Yajugaku-Sasshi, 102, 447-451, May, 1982.

Merchant RE, Andre CA.; A review of recent clinical trials of the nutritional supplement Chlorella pyrenoidosa in the treatment of fibromyalgia, hypertension, and ulcerative colitis. Altern Ther Health Med. 2001 May-Jun;7(3):79-91. Review.

Merchant RE,; Nutritional supplementation with Chlorella pyrenoidosa for mild to moderate hypertension. J Med Food. 2002 Fall;5(3):141-52.

Merchant RE, Carmack CA, Wise CM.; Nutritional supplementation with Chlorella pyrenoidosa for patients with fibromyalgia syndrome: a pilot study. Phytother Res. 2000 May;14(3):167-73.

Merchant, R.E.; Rice, C.C.; Young, H.F.: Dietary Chlorella pyrenoidosa for patients with malignant gl ioma: Effects on immunocompetence, quality of life and survival. Phytotherapy Research, Vol. 4, No. 6, 220-230, 1990.

Miyazawa, Y.; Murayama, T.; Ooya, N.; et al: Immunomodulation by unicellular green algae (Chlorella pyrenoidosa) in tumor-bearing mice. Journal of Ethnopharmacology, 24, 135-146, 1988.

Morimoto T, Nagatsu A.; Anti-tumour-promoting glyceroglycolipids from the green alga, Chlorella vulgaris. Phytochemistry. 1995 Nov;40(5):1433-7.

Murakami, T.: Effect of Heterotrophic Chlorella on Blood Pressure and Development of Apoplexy in Hypertensive Rats. Food Research Inst., Kinku University, Japan.

Murayama, T.: Effect of Various Products Derived from Chlorella Pyrenoidosa Cells on Defense Mechanism of Organism (Immunological Resistance). The 21st Japan Bacteriology Convention, November 1984.

Myers J.; Use of algae for support of the human in space. Life Sci Space Res. 1964;2:323-36.

Noda K, Tanaka K, Yamada A.; Simple assay for antitumour immunoactive glycoprotein derived from Chlorella vulgaris strain CK22 using ELISA. Phytother Res. 2002 Sep;16(6):581-5.

Noda K, Ohno N, Tanaka K, Kamiya N, Okuda M, Yadomae T, Nomoto K, Shoyama Y.; A water-soluble antitumor glycoprotein from Chlorella vulgaris. Planta Med. 1996 Oct;62(5):423-6.

Okamoto K, Iizuka Y.; Effects of Chlorella alkali extract on blood pressure in SHR. Jpn Heart J. 1978 Jul;19(4):622-3.

Otles S, Pire R.; Fatty acid composition of Chlorella and Spirulina microalgae species. J AOAC Int. 2001 Nov-Dec;84(6):1708-14.

Pitchford; Journal of the American Medical Association, 1982, vol. 248; 23. Pitchford, P.; *Healing with Whole Foods* (North Atlantic Books), 2002.

Pore RS.; Detoxification of chlordecone poisoned rats with Chlorella and Chlorella derived sporopollenin. Drug Chem Toxicol. 1984;7(1):57-71.

Price JA 3rd, Sanny C, Shevlin D.; Inhibition of mast cells by algae. J Med Food. 2002 Winter;5(4):205-10.

Pugh N, Ross SA, ElSohly HN, ElSohly MA, Pasco DS.; Isolation of three high molecular weight polysaccharide preparations with potent immunostimulatory activity from Spirulina platensis, aphanizomenon flos-aquae and Chlorella pyrenoidosa. Planta Med. 2001 Nov;67(8):737-42.

Queiroz ML, Rodrigues AP,; Protective effects of Chlorella vulgaris in lead-exposed mice infected with Listeria monocytogenes. Int Immunopharmacol. 2003 Jun;3(6):889-900.

Sakuno, T., et al.: Inhibitory Effect of Chlorella on Increases in Serum and Liver Cho lesterol Levels of Rats. Health Industry Newsletter, March 25, 1 978.

Sano T, Kumamoto Y,; Effect of lipophilic extract of Chlorella vulgaris on alimentary hyperlipidemia in cholesterol-fed rats. Artery. 1988;15(4):217-24.

Sano T, Tanaka Y.; Effect of dried, powdered Chlorella vulgaris on experimental atherosclerosis and alimentary hypercholesterolemia in cholesterol-fed rabbits. Artery. 1987;14(2):76-84.

Shimuzu, M.: Effect of Chlorella on Human Pulse Wave Velocity. Kanazawa Medical University, Dept. of Serology, April 8, 1985.

Singh A, Singh SP, Bamezai R.; Inhibitory potential of Chlorella vulgaris (E-25) on mouse skin papillomagenesis and xenobiotic detoxication system. Anticancer Res. 1999 May-Jun;19(3A):1887-91.

Sponza DT.; Necessity of toxicity assessment in Turkish industrial discharges (examples from metal and textile industry effluents). Environ Monit Assess. 2002 Jan;73(1):41-66.

Steenblock D.; Chlorella, the Natural Medicinal Algae, Physiol Chem, 1956, 305; 182-191.

Tanaka, K.; Koga, T.; Konishi, F.; et al: Augmentation of host defense by a unicellular alga, Chlorella vulgaris, to escherichia coli infection. Infect. Immun., 53, 267-271; 1986.

Tanaka K, Yamada A, Noda K,; A novel glycoprotein obtained from Chlorella vulgaris strain CK22 shows antimetastatic immunopotentiation.Cancer Immunol Immunother. 1998 Feb;45(6):313-20.

Tanaka K, Yamada A, Oral administration of a unicellular green algae, Chlorella vulgaris, prevents stress-induced ulcer. Planta Med. 1997 Oct;63(5):465-6.

Vermeil, C.,: The Stimulation of Tumoricidal Peritoneal Macrophages can be Directly Induced by Peritoneal Implantation of Unicellular Algae in Humans. Arch Inst. Pasteur Tunis. Mar-Jun 62 (1-2) pp. 91-94, 1985.

Want, L.F., Lin, 1.K., Tung, Y.C.: Effect of Chlorella on the levels of glycogen, triglyceride and cholesterol in ethionine treated rats. J. Formosan Medical Assoc., 79 (1), 1-10, 1980.

Wilkinson, S.C.; Goulding, K.H.; Robinson, P.K.: Mercury removal by immobilized algae; (Chlorella) in batch culture systems. Journal of Applied Phycology, 2, 223-230, 1990.

ABOUT THE AUTHOR

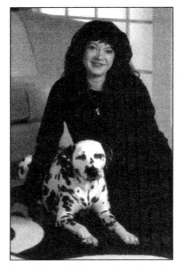

Beth M. Ley, Ph.D., has been a science writer specializing in health and nutrition since 1988 and has written many health-related books, including the best sellers, *DHEA: Unlocking the Secrets to the Fountain of Youth* and *MSM: On Our Way Back to Health With Sulfur*. She wrote her own undergraduate degree program and graduated in Scientific and Technical Writing from North Dakota State University in 1987 (combination of Zoology and Journalism). Beth has her masters (1998) and doctoral degrees (1999) in Nutrition.

Beth also does nutrition and wellness counseling in Detroit Lakes, MN, and speaks on nutrition, health and divine healing locally and nationwide. She is a weekly speaker at Strawberry Lake Christian Retreat, Ogema, MN.

Beth lives in the Minnesota lakes country. She is dedicated to God and to spreading the health message. She enjoys nature and spending time with her dalmatian, KC.

Memberships: New York Academy of Sciences, American Neutraceutical Association, Resurrection Apostolic International Network (RAIN), and Gospel Crusade.

Other Recommended Titles by Beth Ley, Ph.D.

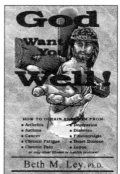

ISBN:1-890766-19-4
240 pages, $14.95

ISBN:0-9642703-0-7
110 pages, $8.95

Credit card orders call toll free:
1-877-BOOKS11
Also visit:
www.blpublications.com

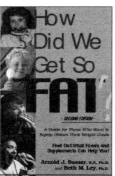

Books from BL Publications

Diabetes to Wholeness!
Beth M. Ley, 120 pgs. $9.95

A natural and spiritual approach to disease prevention and control. Covers Type I and Type II. Learn about significance of whole foods, protective supplements and spiritual roots.

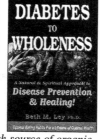

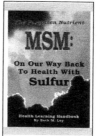

MSM: On Our Way Back To Health With Sulfur Beth M. Ley, 40 pages, $3.95

MSM (methyl sulfonyl methane), is a rich source of organic sulfur, important for connective tissue regeneration. Beneficial for arthritis and other joint problems, allergies, asthma, skin problems, TMJ, periodontal conditions, pain relief, and much more! Includes important "How to use" directions.

How to Fight Osteoporosis & Win: The Miracle of MCHC
Beth M. Ley, 80 pgs. $6.95

Find out if you are at risk for osteoporosis and what to do to prevent and reverse it. Get the truth about bone loss, calcium, supplements, foods, MCHC & much more!

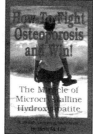

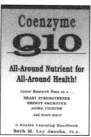

Coenzyme Q10: All Around Nutrient for All-Around Health!
Beth M. Ley-Jacobs, 1999, 60 pages, $4.95

CoQ10 is found in every living cell. With age, insufficient levels become more common, putting us at serious risk of illness and disease. Protect and strengthen the cardiovascular system; benefit blood pressure, immunity, fatigue, weight problems, Alzheimer's, Parkinson's, Huntington's, gum-disease and slow aging.

DHA: The Magnificent Marine Oil
Beth M. Ley-Jacobs, 1999, 120 pages, $6.95

Individuals commonly lack this essential Omega-3 fatty acid so important to the brain, vision, and immune system and much more. Memory, depression, ADD, addiction disorders, inflammatory disorders, skin problems, schizophrenia, elevated blood lipids, etc., benefit from DHA.

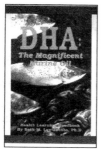

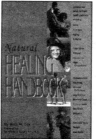

Natural Healing Handbook
Beth M. Ley, 320 pgs.$14.95

Excellent, easy -to-use reference book with natural health care remedies for all your healthcare concerns. A book you will use over & over again!

TO PLACE AN ORDER:

___ *Aspirin Alternatives: The Top Natural Pain-Relieving Analgesics* (Lombardi) $8.95

___ *Bilberry & Lutein: The Vision Enhancers!* (Ley) $4.95

___ *Calcium: The Facts, Fossilized Coral* (Ley) $4.95

___ *Castor Oil: Its Healing Properties* (Ley) $4.95

___ *Chlorella: The Ultimate Green Food* (Ley) $4.95

___ *Dr. John Willard on Catalyst Altered Water* (Ley) $3.95

___ *CoQ10: All-Around Nutrient for All-Around Health* (Ley) .. $4.95

___ *Colostrum: Nature's Gift to the Immune System* (Ley) $5.95

___ *DHA: The Magnificent Marine Oil* (Ley) $6.95

___ *DHEA: Unlocking the Secrets of the Fountain of Youth - 2nd Edition* (Ash & Ley)...................................$14.95

___ *Diabetes to Wholeness* (Ley) $9.95

___ *Discover the Beta Glucan Secret* (Ley) $3.95

___ *Fading: One family's journey with a women silenced by Alzheimer's* (Kraft) $12.95

___ *Flax! Fabulous Flax!* (Ley) $4.95

___ *God Wants You Well* (Ley) $14.95

___ *Health Benefits of Probiotics* (Dash) $4.95

___ *How Did We Get So Fat? 2nd Edition* (Susser & Ley) $8.95

___ *How to Fight Osteoporosis and Win!* (Ley) $6.95

___ *Maca: Adaptogen and Hormonal Regulator* (Ley) $4.95

___ *Marvelous Memory Boosters* (Ley) $3.95

___ *Medicinal Mushrooms: Agaricus Blazei Murill* (Ley) $4.95

___ *MSM: On Our Way Back to Health W/ Sulfur* (Ley) SPANISH $3.95

___ *MSM: On Our Way Back to Health w/ Sulfur* (Ley) $3.95

___ *Natural Healing Handbook* (Ley) $14.95

___ *Nature's Road to Recovery: Nutritional Supplements for the Alcoholic & Chemical Dependent* (Ley) $5.95

___ *PhytoNutrients: Medicinal Nutrients Found in Foods* (Ley) $3.95

___ *The Potato Antioxidant: Alpha Lipoic Acid* (Ley) $6.95

___ *Vinpocetine: Revitalize Your Brain w/ Periwinkle Extract!* (Ley) $4.95

Subtotal $ _____Please add $4.00 for shipping **TOTAL $**_____

Send check or money order to:
BL Publications 14325 Barnes Drive Detroit Lakes, MN 56501
Credit card orders call toll free: 1-877-BOOKS11
or visit: www.blpublications.com